T0144852

BASIC HEALTH PUBLICATIONS USER'S GUIDE

TO HERBAL REMEDIES

Learn About the Most Popular Herbs for Preventing Disease and Staying Healthy.

HYLA CASS, M.D.

JACK CHALLEM Series Editor

The information contained in this book is based upon the research and personal and professional experiences of the author. It is not intended as a substitute for consulting with your physician or other healthcare provider. Any attempt to diagnose and treat an illness should be done under the direction of a healthcare professional.

The publisher does not advocate the use of any particular healthcare protocol but believes the information in this book should be available to the public. The publisher and author are not responsible for any adverse effects or consequences resulting from the use of the suggestions, preparations, or procedures discussed in this book. Should the reader have any questions concerning the appropriateness of any procedures or preparations mentioned, the author and the publisher strongly suggest consulting a professional healthcare advisor.

Series Editor: Jack Challem
Editor: Christopher Mariadason
Typesetter: Gary A. Rosenberg
Series Cover Designer: Mike Stromberg

Basic Health Publications User's Guides are published by Basic Health Publications, Inc.

ISBN: 978-1-59120-088-8 (Pbk.)
ISBN: 978-1-68162-859-2 (Hardcover)

CONTENTS

INTRODUCTION

People in every culture and every country have been using herbs as natural remedies for thousands of years. Safe and effective, herbs have passed the test of time and have helped millions of people maintain or recover their health. Today, they are being used by increasing numbers of people seeking natural alternatives to synthetic and often hazardous drugs.

It may seem strange that modern drugs can be replaced with grandma's teas, powders, and tinctures. But extensive scientific evidence supports the use of herbal medicines, and many modern drugs are actually synthetic versions of substances found in plants. In the United States, the medical profession is slowly beginning to catch on to this, despite having dismissed the value of herbs in the past, preferring to prescribe expensive drugs instead. In contrast, European doctors have always maintained their interest and skill in prescribing herbal medicines, or phytomedicines, in conjunction with pharmaceuticals. Europe has a stronger history of herb use compared with the United States, and, not surprisingly, most of the scientific research on herbs has been conducted there.

Why use herbs instead of synthetic medications? The fact is, herbs possess many properties that make them superior to synthetic drugs in many ways, including being more in tune with the body and, therefore, creating fewer, and certainly less harmful, side effects. Moreover, most herbs have multiple uses, bestowing *side benefits* instead of side effects. For example, ginkgo not only improves memory, but can also boost blood circulation to the arms and legs. And garlic not only enhances the immune system, but lowers cholesterol as well. In addition, many herbs fulfill roles that drugs cannot. To wit, milk thistle, when administered early enough, can protect the liver from mushroom poisoning. And the whole range of adaptogens have no equivalent in the world of conventional medication.

Herbs are also appealing in that they can be purchased without a prescription, are relatively inexpensive, and are quite safe when used as directed. In this *User's Guide to Herbal Remedies*, you will learn what herbs are, how they work, and how to buy and use them. You will find detailed descriptions of ten of the most popular herbal medicines. Whether you're young or old, male or female, you will learn how to use herbs to improve your health and well-being.

CHAPTER 1

HERBAL MEDICINE: FROM FOLKLORE TO SCIENCE

The use of herbs is as old as human history. From the most primitive jungle-dwellers to the highly sophisticated Chinese and Indians, every culture has had its herbal remedies. Traditional Chinese medicine (TCM) and Ayurveda (East Indian) are two important ancient healing systems that have not only withstood the test of time, but are gaining new respect based on current research findings. Both systems use specific herbs native to their geographical area, and often in specific combinations designed to treat a multitude of conditions. Both the Chinese and Ayurvedic systems are comprehensive, treating the body and mind as an interacting unit.

The Growing Popularity of Herbs

A medicinal herb is any plant that can benefit one's health. The end-product can be derived from various parts of the plant— the leaf, as in ginkgo, the fruit, as in saw palmetto, or the root, as in ginseng. Rich in vitamins, minerals, and vitamin-like compounds such as polyphenols, flavo - noids, and carotenoids, these products are used by the body to enhance its multitude of biochemical processes.

About 80 percent of the world's population uses herbal medicines, from the most basic folk remedies to the well-researched phytomedicines of Europe and Asia. Doctors who are given the choice between prescribing herbs or pharmaceuticals often make herbs their first choice. For example, in Germany, doctors have prescribed St. John's wort, an herb used to treat depression, twenty times as often as the leading antidepressant drug. Why? Because the herb is just as effective, it costs less, and it does not have the negative side effects of the drug.

Sales of botanical products in the United States are also growing, and now exceed $4 billion annually. Of course this is just a fraction of the annual sales of all pharmaceuticals, which amounts to between $50 billion and $60 billion a year. In a 1998 study, Hartman and New Hope surveyed 43,442 American households and found that 68 percent had consumed a vitamin, mineral, or herbal supplement in the previous six months. Despite this growing acceptance of herbs, North America still lags far behind Europe in both herb use and research.

Western Medicine vs. Herbal Healing

Unlike Western medicine, traditional herbal medical practitioners tailor each diagnosis and treatment to fit the individual. This certainly makes sense when you consider that, from our faces to our fingerprints, no two of us are exactly alike. When designing a treatment, herbal practitioners pay special attention to every aspect of the individual, aiming at building health and not just covering up a specific ailment.

Another important difference is that traditional medicine practitioners look beyond just the chemical and molecular components of herbs, focusing as well on their *energetic* aspects. What does this mean? Unlike manufactured drugs, the healing powers of herbs are likely due to more than just the molecules involved! The energy field of the plant meeting the energy field of the individual may produce an additional healing influence. This concept appears not only in Eastern medicine, but in Native American beliefs as well, where the *spirit* (in effect, the energy) of an herb is directly involved in the battle with illness.

While this concept may sound strange to our Western mindset, it can be explained scientifically. All living things, from plants to humans, contain energy. In order to grow, plants must first absorb energy from the sun and transform it. When we ingest plants, our body takes in the energy of a given plant and uses it to sustain us. The chemicals in our bodies are basically shells that carry energy. The Chinese call our vital energy force *qi*. Whereas Western medicine is concerned with fighting the illness itself, Chinese medicine views illness as a blockage of this vital life force. When we are ill, it may be the result of a blockage of our ability to access and utilize our full energy potential.

We can begin to understand this concept by looking at the success of acupuncture, which is based on unblocking flow along the unseen energy pathways of the body called *meridians*. As an analogy, consider a flowing river, full of energy and life. If we dam the river and block its flow, the water turns stagnant and fills with mosquitoes. Now we can the fix this problem with toxic pesticides that kill the mosquitoes, but that would also hurt the fish, as well as anyone who drank the water. A better alternative would be to release the blockage (open the dam) to allow the water to flow freely again, forcing the mosquitoes to leave. Similarly, during illness, if our energy flow is blocked, all it may take is the right herb to open the blockage to allow the body's energy to flow, thus enabling the healing processes.

How Herbs Differ from Pharmaceuticals

Many people don't realize that herbs are the original source of at least 25 percent of all pharmaceuticals. Often drugs either are made from, or are synthetic duplicates of, chemicals originally isolated from healing plants. Some examples are morphine, a potent painkiller, which comes from the opium poppy; digitalis, a cardiac stimulant, which comes from foxglove; and reserpine, a sedative and antihypertensive, which comes from rauwolfia (Indian snakeroot).

Herbs generally work with your own body processes to fight off disease. For example, echinacea increases the activity of your infection-fighting white blood cells. And milk thistle enhances the liver's production of the antioxidant glutathione to fight free radicals. Unlike Western medicine, which looks for the active ingredients in a plant and then extracts it, discarding the rest of the plant, herbal medicine relies on the synergistic action of the whole plant, which may contain thousands of compounds. Most often, an herbal medicine made from the whole plant is more effective than its separate, isolated ingre - dients because these compounds work in concert to promote health. Herbs also tend to work more gradually, helping to strengthen the body's defenses over time. Drugs, on the other hand, have a more rapid and targeted action, which is also why they are also more likely to cause side effects.

Safety of Herbs

When comparing the safety of herbs to that of synthetic drugs, we must note a recent study that showed there are as many as 100,000 deaths in hospitals a year from the use of pre-scribed drugs, *used as directed,* and more than 2 million serious reactions annually to prescription drugs. In contrast, deaths from herbal medicines are extremely rare. While there has been some negative publicity about ephedra, an herb used to promote weight loss, the truth is that the deaths attributed to it may have been due to various other causes, and that the herb itself had a minor role if any at all. Of course all herbs must be used responsibly, and in the case of ephedra, individuals with weakened hearts should not use it at all, especially when combined with the synthetic ephedrine, an ingredient in common cold remedies that is a known cardiac stimulant.

The most common negative reactions to herbs are allergic symptoms such as rashes and upset stomachs. Negative reactions to herbs, as to drugs, may be idiosyncratic, and not on the usual "side effects" list. We each have our unique biochemistry and our own reactions. I warn my patients that if they feel any ill effects from an herb they are using, they should trust this response and immediately reduce the dose or simply stop taking it, and see if that makes a difference. In any case, if one herb causes a problem there are always others that can be taken instead.

Using Herbs Sensibly:
Drug-Herb Interactions

Generally speaking, people taking prescription medicines can safely use most herbs, but I recommend checking with your doctor before treating the same condition with both a drug and an herb. Since most doctors are not well–versed in this issue, they are most likely to tell you to stop the herb. This should not, however, dissuade you from revealing this to him or her, since there can be serious side effects from drug-herb interactions.

One example of a contraindicated combination is St. John's wort with a monoamine oxidase (MAO)–inhibiting antidepressant, or with a variety of other drugs such as coumadin and cyclosporine. Another is ginkgo, which acts as a blood thinner, with any other blood thinner (anticoagulant). For more specific information on this subject, see *Herb Contraindications and Drug Interactions* by Francis Brinker and Nancy Stodart, as well as several websites, such as supplementinfo.org.

There are some positive drug-herb combinations as well, some of which I routinely prescribe for my patients. For example, those taking a drug that is metabolized by the liver, such as an antidepressant, are given milk thistle, an herb that supports normal liver function. And I recommend echinacea after a course of antibiotics in order to strengthen the immune system.

Herbs, Pregnancy, and Children

Women have to be cautious about their herbal intake during pregnancy and while nursing, since any herbs they take can also affect the baby. Many herbs have not been approved for use during pregnancy and nursing. A good source for this information is the authoritative German Commission E Monograph.

German Commission E Monograph *A collection of reports on herb safety and efficacy, written by researchers and clinicians in Germany for that country's equivalent of the U.S. FDA.*

In many cases, herbs may be the preferred treatment for children, but it is important to follow sound advice when adjusting the dosages. In general, the adult dosages should be adjusted in accordance with the child's weight. An excellent resource is *Smart Medicine for a Healthier Child: A Practical A-to-Z Reference to Natural and Conventional Treatments for Infants & Children*, by

Janet Zand, Rachel Walton, and Bob Rountree. The easiest form for a child to take is a liquid, especially one with a glycerin base, which is sweet. If you prefer the more potent alcohol tinctures, you can simply add it to hot water to evaporate the alcohol. Then, you can disguise the taste by mixing the liquid with applesauce, yogurt, or mashed potatoes.

The New Science of Herbs

Research studies are the backbone of conventional medicine and provide a wealth of valuable information in all fields, including human biology and the health sciences. Since the demand for a more natural approach to medicine, including the use of herbs, is increasing in North America, there is an increasing interest in research. But the issue of herbal research in the United States has been complicated by important non-scientific factors that influence which therapies receive funding. Research is costly, running into the millions, and most natural products do not have any major funding to support them.

In the United States, pharmaceutical companies will choose to bear the cost of research on a natural product only if they are sure they can obtain a patent for any new products that result from their investment. And therein lies a major problem, since, for the most part, natural products like herbs are not easily patented, and any research on them belongs in the public domain, regardless of who is paying for it. And if companies can't maintain exclusive control of the research they paid for, they're obviously reluctant to invest in herbal studies that might also aid their competitors.

As a result of the drug companies' tremendous investments in their products, and of their collaboration with medical schools for research purposes, much of the information taught to doctors in medical school and beyond comes from the industry itself. In Europe—where many herbal medicines are classified alongside pharmaceutical drugs, prescribed by doctors, and covered by the national health plans—it's a different story. Because herbal medicine is accepted in Europe as a legitimate form of therapy, their drug companies have the financial incentive to do the necessary research.

It is likely that the American pharmaceutical industry will follow the European lead and create refined extracts, which can be patented. Unfortunately, this approach involves focusing on the so-called active ingredients and removing the so-called "extraneous" materials that actually add to the herbs' power, effectiveness, and safety. Since existing herbal research is pointing in the direction of whole extracts, this approach may be continued in the United States. There is still a great deal of discussion about this issue and other topics regarding how best to extract, standardize, and provide herbal products. In the meantime, however, we will have to be careful that herbs do not become solely prescription items, thereby restricting their use.

Working with Your Doctor

In the best of all possible worlds, your doctor would be familiar with herbal remedies and would prescribe them as needed. I believe most doctors are motivated to find the best, least harmful approaches to helping their patients. I therefore recommend that you take this book or something similar to your doctor to introduce him to the benefits of herbal medicine. He may be skeptical, but draw his attention to the scientific references at the back of the book and encourage him in a non-argumentative way to look them up and read them. Sharing this knowledge can help you, your doctor, and his or her other patients.

Remember, there are times when it's important to seek professional medical help—for example, in cases of high blood pressure, liver ailment, enlarged prostate, severe depression, or deteriorating mental function. All are potentially serious conditions and should be carefully evaluated before you embark on a self-treatment program.

CHAPTER 2

ECHINACEA—
IMMUNE ENHANCER

*E*chinacea (ek-i-NAY-sha) *purpurea*, also known as the purple coneflower, is one of the most popular herbal medications in the world. For more than a century, millions of people in the United States and Europe have regularly taken echinacea at the first sign of a cold or the flu. Traditional Native American tribal healers used a related species, *Echinacea angustifolia*, to treat a wide variety of problems, including respiratory infection, inflammation of the eyes, toothache, and snakebite. And prior to the advent of sulfa drugs in the 1930s, echinacea was the leading cold and flu remedy in the United States.

In Germany, echinacea is the primary remedy for minor respiratory infections, with more than 1.3 million prescriptions written annually. Echinacea is also used to treat ear infections, bronchitis, bladder infections, and even yeast infections. Unlike antibiotics, which are of little benefit for treating these types of infections, echinacea can greatly reduce many annoying and painful symptoms.

How Echinacea Works

Echinacea enhances the immune system, the complex combination of responses that fights invaders such as bacteria and viruses. The immune system fights infections by producing antibodies, which are specific molecules made by blood cells in response to a specific antigen, or invader. The next time these antibodies encounter these antigens, they recognize them and fight them off. Without the immune system, we would succumb to every infective agent we encounter.

Echinacea stimulates antibody production, raises the white blood cell count, and stimulates the activity of the white blood cells that fight infection. These white blood cells include lymphocytes, which fight viruses; natural killer cells, which attack tumor cells; and macrophages, which gobble up disease-causing

Lymphocytes
Small white blood cells that carry out the activities of the immune system.

bacteria. The two major classes of lymphocytes are B cells, which grow to maturity independent of the thymus, and T cells, which are processed in the thymus.

Scientific Evidence

There are more than 400 published studies on echinacea, with 11 consisting of especially well controlled double-blind studies. One of these followed 108 patients with acute flu-like illnesses. Half of the patients were given echinacea, and the other half were given a placebo (dummy pill). After eight weeks, the results showed that the treated group stayed healthier longer, and the people from that group who did get sick had shorter, less severe illnesses.

Another double-blind study of echinacea examined its effects on flu-like illnesses. Researchers studied 180 flu sufferers who were divided into three groups. One group was given a placebo, another group 450 mg of echinacea, and the third group 900 mg of echinacea daily. By the third day, the

Double-Blind Study
A study in which neither test subjects nor investigators know which subjects are receiving the active substance.

subjects receiving the higher dose of echinacea showed significant reductions in flu symptoms, which included chills, sweating, sore throat, muscle ache, and headache. There was no improvement in the other two groups. In addition to demonstrating the effectiveness of echinacea, this study also highlighted the importance of taking an adequate dose.

Echinacea and Yeast Infections

Hard-to-treat, recurring yeast infections often yield to echinacea. In one study, researchers treated 203 women suffering from chronic vaginal yeast infections with either oral doses of echinacea or a topical antifungal cream medication. The herbal group did 3.5 times better than the medicated group. Only 16.7 percent of the echinacea group had a recurrence of the infection, as opposed to 60.5 percent of the medicated group. Echinacea also boosted the women's overall immunity. Since recurrent yeast infections can be bothersome, to say the least, and do not always respond to conventional treatment, this is a significant finding. It illustrates how supporting the immune system, rather than simply treating the symptom, enhances recovery for the patient.

Echinacea and Children

As we all know, once children start day care or school, they often pick up colds, flus, and ear infections. This is natural, given the close proximity to other children and an immature immune system that doesn't yet recognize many common pathogens. An excellent preventive measure during the cold and flu season is a daily dosage of echinacea. Children prefer a glycerin-based tincture or a tea, which can be given two to three times a day. A two-day break is recommended every eight weeks. One of my patients brought in her five-year-old son, who had been catching every bug that came to school, and then passing it on to her. I suggested the glycerin-based tincture for him and the alcohol-based tincture for his mother. Both remained free of illness for the rest of the season!

Safety and Dosages

Echinacea has been shown to be very safe, even when taken in extremely high doses. Side effects are rare and are usually limited to minor gastrointestinal symptoms, increased urination, or a mild allergic reaction.

The typical daily dose of powdered echinacea extract is 300 mg, taken three times a day. Alcohol tinctures containing one part echinacea to five parts alcohol are usually taken at a dose of 3 to 4 ml three times daily; echinacea juice at a dose of 2 to 3 ml three times daily; and whole dried root at 1 to 2 grams three times daily. Echinacea is usually taken at the first sign of a cold and continued for seven to fourteen days. It can also be taken continuously for prevention, with two days off every two months. This break is recommended so that the body does not become too accustomed to the echinacea, leading to a reduction in efficacy.

Choosing an Echinacea Supplement

Many herbalists feel that the liquid forms of echinacea are more effective than the tablets or capsules. Some believe that part of echinacea's benefit may be due to direct contact with the tonsils. The liquid forms may also contain more of the active ingredients, or possibly the ingredients are in a form that is more easily absorbed.

Echinacea is also frequently combined with goldenseal (*Hydrastis canadensis*) in cold prepa-

rations. The prime ingredient of goldenseal, ber-
berine, appears to activate the white blood cells.

Cautions

Germany's Commission E warns against using
echinacea in cases of tuberculosis or in autoimmune disorder, such as multiple sclerosis (MS) or
lupus. These warnings are based on fears that
echinacea might actually overstimulate immunity.
There are also warnings that echinacea should
not be used by persons with acquired immune
deficiency syndrome (AIDS). Low doses can be
used in the early stages to treat any accompany-
ing infections, but not in more advanced stages.
Echinacea *is* safe for pregnant women. There are
no known drug interactions.

I have been recommending echinacea to my
patients and family and have used it myself for
years. And while using this powerful herb doesn't
guarantee that you will never catch a cold, when
used correctly, echinacea can help to ward off
infection and shorten both the length and severity of illnesses. The point is that while echinacea
is not a quick fix, used correctly over time, it can
increase your natural resistance to bacterial, fungal, and viral infections.

CHAPTER 3

GARLIC—
CARDIOVASCULAR
AND IMMUNE-SYSTEM
BOOSTER

Humans have cultivated garlic (*Allium sativum*) for at least 5,000 years, and today this herbal medicine is found almost everywhere in the world, from Polynesia to Siberia. By the end of the first century A.D., Dioscorides, Hippocrates, and other ancient Greek physicians recommended garlic for many conditions, including respiratory problems, parasites, and poor digestion. Garlic is principally used now to prevent and treat heart disease, hardening of the arteries, high blood pressure, and high levels of cholesterol and triglycerides. The primary active ingredient in garlic is allicin, a sulfur-containing compound that the body converts into other therapeutic compounds. Allicin is found only in garlic products produced by crushing the fresh bulb, not in those produced by steam distillation of the oil.

Reversing Heart Disease

Garlic has been shown to be helpful in preventing and reversing atherosclerosis—the dangerous hardening of the arteries that causes high blood pressure, heart disease, and stroke. The evidence for using garlic to treat atherosclerosis comes from numerous animal and human studies. Garlic has been shown to reduce the size of plaque deposits, the "hard" material that clogs and stiffens arteries, by nearly 50 percent in humans, rats, and rabbits. And in a recent study of 200 men and women conducted over a two-year period, those who took 300 mg or more of garlic daily showed improvement in the flexibility of their aorta, the main artery that carries blood from the heart. Garlic extracts have also been shown to reduce blood pressure in dogs and rats, and numerous animal studies have shown that it can reduce blood clotting. Taken as a whole, this makes garlic a remarkably effective treatment for arterial disease.

Plaque
"Hard" material deposited in the walls of arteries, causing them to clog and stiffen, leading to high blood pressure, heart disease, and stroke.

Garlic Reduces Cholesterol

High blood levels of cholesterol and other lipids (fats), such as triglycerides, are related to a higher incidence of heart disease. Thus, physicians recommend keeping cholesterol and triglyceride levels down. Especially important to control is the form of cholesterol known as low-density lipoprotein (LDL), the so-called "bad" cholesterol that damages arteries. It is also important that when lowering our LDL levels we maintain a good ratio of another form of cholesterol, called high-density lipoprotein (HDL), which is a "good" form that actually protects our arteries.

Triglycerides
Derived from fats in foods or made in the body, triglycerides, together with cholesterol, form the plasma lipids or fats in the blood.

At least twenty-eight controlled clinical studies (studies in which its effects are compared with those of a placebo and/or a drug) have shown that garlic lowers total cholesterol levels by between 9 and 12 percent, while improving the important ratio of good to bad cholesterol. In one German study conducted in 1990, 261 patients received either 800 mg of standardized garlic or a placebo daily. Over the course of sixteen weeks, patients in the garlic group had a 12 percent drop in their total cholesterol and a 17 percent decrease in their triglyceride levels.

Another European study found that garlic was just as effective as the prescription drug Bezafibrate for lowering cholesterol, without any of the drug's side effects. Like prescription drugs, garlic appears to work by interfering with the body's ability to manufacture cholesterol. While not every garlic study has shown the same level of benefit, the reason for inconsistent outcomes is believed to be differences in the manufacturing of particular types of garlic.

A "Natural" Antibiotic

Numerous studies, some dating back to the 1940s, have found that garlic has powerful antibiotic and antiviral properties. Persons infected with the human immunodeficiency virus (HIV) have taken garlic to prevent secondary bacterial and yeast infections, a use based on sound scientific research. Garlic has also been used to treat certain viral and fungal infections, including intestinal, oral, and vaginal candida. Noted physician Albert Schweitzer, MD, gave garlic to treat amoebic dysentery in Africa. These antibiotic benefits are most effective when using either raw garlic or a preparation with an allicin content that is the equivalent of raw garlic.

Recently, scientists in Ethiopia tested the antibacterial power of two concentrations (high and low) of garlic extracts against a number of common bacteria that cause pneumonia, including *Streptococcus pneumoniae* and *Klebsiella pneumoniae*. Their study found that both the high and low garlic concentrations triggered an 88 percent response rate, meaning garlic clearly inhibited the growth of both organisms, leading the researchers to conclude that garlic could be used as an effective antibacterial agent for these pathogenic microorganisms.

Another team of researchers has also revealed equally promising results in a second study that tested allicin against an antibiotic-resistant bacterium called VRE *(vancomycin-resistant enterococcus)*. The allicin stopped the growth and proliferation of VRE in cell culture experiments, which showed that allicin could inhibit the bacteria. The researchers suggested that individuals at high risk for antibiotic-resistant infections—such as people with impaired immunity or those who are about to enter a germ-rich hospital environment—could use garlic supplements to prevent infections.

When researchers from the University of Toronto exposed cultured, malaria-infected human cells to a mixture of disulfides, which are compounds found in garlic, they reported that it quickly killed the malaria parasites. The authors of the study believe that the garlic ingredients interfered with a key enzyme that allows the malaria parasites to infect human blood.

Garlic's Anticancer Effects

The same team of Canadian researchers involved in the malaria study also revealed that garlic disulfide compounds are equally effective at protecting humans from cultured melanoma (cancer) cells. Researchers speculate that the same enzyme involved in the spread of malaria in human blood cells is involved in encouraging cancer cells to reproduce. Garlic was shown in this study to interfere with this enzyme, thereby halting the spread of melanoma.

Several other large studies have strongly suggested that diets high in garlic can prevent cancer, especially cancers of the colon, esophagus, and stomach. In one 1986 study, a group of 41,837 women were questioned about their lifestyle habits. Four years later, follow-up questionnaires revealed that those women whose diet included a significant amount of garlic were approximately 30 percent less likely to develop colon cancer.

Another recent study has shown that garlic can cut the risk of prostate cancer. Researchers surveyed the eating habits of 238 men with prostate cancer and 471 healthy controls in Shanghai, China. They found that the risk of prostate cancer declined by more than 33 percent in men who consumed small amounts of onions, garlic, scallions, shallots, and leeks each day. Garlic proved to be a particularly potent anticancer agent: Men who consumed 2 grams of garlic daily experienced a 50 percent decease in prostate can - cer risk. Even eating one clove of garlic a day appeared to provide protection against cancer. That is certainly another good reason for you to eat your garlic!

Choosing a Garlic Supplement

Eating one or two cloves of raw garlic a day should be sufficient for most health benefits, but many people choose to avoid eating raw garlic because of possible negative social aftereffects. For this reason, some companies sell odorless substitutes made from the allicin in garlic. There are also enteric-coated garlic powder supplements. (The enteric coating delays digestion of the tablet until it passes from the stomach to the intestines.) For health maintenance, 2,500 mcg of allicin daily is enough, while for therapeutic purposes, at least 5,000 mcg of allicin a day is necessary. You could also encourage your family and friends to eat garlic. This way, no one will notice your breath!

Safety and Dosages

The only common side effect that results from taking garlic is the characteristic unpleasant breath odor. Even taking an odorless supplement offers no protection, since this form produces an offensive smell in up to 50 percent of users. Other side effects, such as nausea, headache, sweating, and dizziness, occur only rarely.

Cautions

Raw garlic, taken in excessive doses, can cause numerous symptoms, such as heartburn, nausea, stomach upset, vomiting, diarrhea, flatulence, facial flushing, rapid pulse, and insomnia. When applied to the skin, garlic can also lead to skin irritation, blistering, and even burns.

Since garlic thins the blood, it would be prudent to avoid taking high-potency garlic pills prior to surgery or if you are already taking prescription blood thinners. However, garlic is presumed to be safe for pregnant and nursing women. Nursing babies actually seem to like the taste.

CHAPTER 4

GINKGO—MEMORY AND CIRCULATION ENHANCER

If one were to search for a natural compound that could offer protective benefits against the effects of aging, surely ginkgo would appear to be a most likely candidate. *Ginkgo biloba*, or ginkgo, as it's commonly known, is the most widely prescribed herb in Germany, with more than 6 million prescriptions being written in a typical year. Used primarily to treat failing mental faculties, including memory loss in the elderly, ginkgo is also used to treat a variety of circulatory problems.

More than 200 million years old, ginkgo is the oldest surviving species of tree on the planet. Moreover, individual trees may live for up to one thousand years! The bilobed—that is, double lobed—leaf gives the plant the name "biloba." The active ingredients responsible for ginkgo's health benefits are two unique compounds called flavone glycosides and ginkgolides. Nearly all research on ginkgo is done using a leaf extract standardized to 24-percent flavone gly-cosides and 6-percent ginkgolides. These substances are potent antioxidants, somewhat similar to flavonoids found in fruits and vegetables, that bind to free radicals to render them harmless and prevent cellular damage.

Ginkgo as an Antioxidant

A leading source of illness and aging are free

radicals, which are unstable molecules that damage cells and even their DNA or genetic content. These dangerous free radicals are both a normal byproduct of our metabolism, and increasingly, products of toxins such as cigarette smoke, car exhaust, pesticides, and other chemicals in our air, food, and water. They can, however, be neutralized by *antioxidants,* which are compounds that bind to the free radicals, making them harmless. Many plants, ginkgo included, have antioxidant properties built in to protect themselves from the ravages of nature, such as intense sunlight, drought, and pests. The antioxidant properties of ginkgo likely consist of one mechanism by which it protects the brain, the blood vessels, and the circulatory system in general.

Ginkgo and Alzheimer's Disease

Often prescribed for elderly people suffering from impaired mental function (dementia), caused by Alzheimer's disease and impaired circulation to the brain, ginkgo has been found to enhance cerebral blood circulation and flow of oxygen.

Alzheimer's disease (also called "senile dementia of the Alzheimer type") is a chronic and progressive degenerative neurological condition that currently afflicts more than four million people in the United States, and accounts for up to 60 percent of all cases of dementia. Alzheimer's commonly appears after age fifty, and from age sixty-five on, the risk of developing the disease doubles every subsequent five years.

A review of more than forty double-blind controlled studies published in the respected medical journal *The Lancet* concluded that ginkgo extract is an effective treatment for dementia. Researchers have found that ginkgo can be especially helpful when given to patients at the first sign of symptoms. In one published study, German scientists gave a daily dose of 120 mg of ginkgo to twenty elderly patients exhibiting various early symptoms of dementia. The results were dramatic, and the patients receiving ginkgo showed impressive improvements on a variety of clinical tests, as compared with the other patients receiving a placebo (dummy pill).

In one large study published in 1996, German researchers tested ginkgo extract on a group of 222 patients, aged fifty-five or older, who were diagnosed with mild to moderate dementia caused by either Alzheimer's disease or multi-infarct dementia. Patients were given either 240 mg of *Ginkgo biloba* extract twice a day before meals or a placebo for the duration of the six-month long trial. At the conclusion of the study, the researchers reported that patients receiving ginkgo showed a remarkable overall improvement in their condition, including a 300 percent increase in memory and attention as compared with those receiving the placebo pills. The researchers concluded their report by stating that, in cases of dementia, ginkgo extract could improve a patient's quality of life while preserving their independence and postponing the need for (and expense of) full-time care.

A 1997 study by Le Bars published in the *Journal of the American Medical Association* (*JAMA*) reported on the results of a year-long double-blind trial of ginkgo's effect on mental function. More than 300 patients were given either 40 mg of ginkgo extract or a placebo three times daily. The patients taking the ginkgo improved in varying degrees, some quite significantly. What is perhaps more important is the fact that most of them did not follow the usual course of continued deterioration of mental functioning, while most of those receiving the placebo did.

In 2002, researchers at the Cochrane Collaboration at Oxford University in England reviewed and evaluated human clinical trials on standardized concentrated extracts of ginkgo leaf. The researchers focused on thirty-three clinical studies that it considered of acceptable design, size, and quality; all of which lasted from three to fifty-two weeks, with most being twelve weeks. The group concluded that the herbal extract "appears to be safe in use with no excessive side effects," and "there is promising evidence of improvement in cognition and function associated with Ginkgo."

Ginkgo and Memory in Healthy Older Adults

In evaluating media coverage on any scientific research, you must realize that the media often takes information out of context and may make the issues black and white for maximum impact. Here is a classic example of this: A study published in the *Journal of the American Medical Association* in 2002 by Solomon and colleagues concluded that ginkgo does *not* enhance memory or improve cognitive ability in healthy adults over age sixty. The six-week placebo-controlled study tested healthy adults for learning, memory, attention, concentration, and verbal fluency using the standard dose of 120 mg of ginkgo extract per day.

The truth is, not only were there a number of flaws in the study, but ginkgo, in fact, *has* been established as a valuable treatment for dementia, and there has been evidence of its success with healthy older adults. A similar study by Mix and Crews published in *Human Psychopharmacology* in 2002 using a similar population but a higher dosage (180 mg per day) of ginkgo showed significant benefits to memory and other mental abilities. Unfortunately, the average reader might skim the headlines and accept the fact that ginkgo does not work for any type of memory impairment. The loss is to the public, particularly the individuals who would stand to benefit from taking this proven remedy.

Ginkgo Improves Performance of Younger Brains

Several studies have shown that ginkgo helps brain function in younger people as well, by increasing the blood flow in the brain—that is, by improving how well the brain's cells are nourished. Students who use ginkgo in the morning just before going to school to take an examination find a noticeable improvement in their ability to recall information. It appears to work better for this purpose when taken as a loading dose just before it's needed than when taken long-term. This enhancement of young people's short-term memory and concentration has been confirmed by electroencephalogram (EEG) brainwave testing, as well.

Ginkgo and Depression

Ginkgo appears to improve depression, a serious problem that affects more than 17 million Americans. When German researchers treated forty depressed patients with 80 mg of ginkgo three times a day, they reported a 68 percent reduction in the severity of depression after eight weeks. Overall the patients were significantly happier, more optimistic, and more motivated. As a result of the impressive effects ginkgo has on depression, the German Ministry of Health Committee for Herbal Remedies has approved the use of ginkgo extract for improving mood and mental processes.

Ginkgo Enhances Blood Flow

Ginkgo protects and improves the overall performance of the circulatory system. One of the greatest health benefits of ginkgo is its ability to increase blood flow—and oxygen delivery—throughout the entire body, both through its effects on the blood vessels themselves and its actions on platelet-activating factor (PAF). It has also been shown to be effective in strengthening weakened blood vessels, while restoring some of the elasticity that veins commonly lose with age.

A number of animal and human studies have shown that ginkgo is more effective than many standard drugs in relaxing arteries and improving blood circulation. In one human trial, researchers compared ginkgo with standard drugs used to treat vasoconstriction (constriction of the blood vessels). Twenty-five patients were treated with ginkgo and compared with 300 other patients receiving standard medications. By measuring the increase in arteriolar dilation in the big toe of volunteers, the researchers determined that the standard drugs resulted in a 39 percent increase in artery dilation, compared with a 44 percent increase in the group receiving ginkgo.

Ginkgo and Intermittent Claudication

Additional benefits related to ginkgo's ability to increase blood flow include relieving a condition called *intermittent claudication.* This disabling and hard-to-treat leg pain is caused by thick deposits of plaque in the peripheral arteries. After about six weeks of treatment with ginkgo, there is often a marked improvement. According to the Commission E Monographs, at least four double-blind studies have shown that ginkgo can increase the pain-free walking distance by about 75 to 500 feet. Both Germany and the World Health Organization have approved ginkgo use as recognized treatment for this and related conditions.

Ginkgo Inhibits PAF

Another way that ginkgo helps to increase circulation is by inhibiting PAF (platelet-activating factor), a compound that normally helps the body form clots to minimize blood loss from wounds. Unfortunately, excessively elevated levels of PAF cause blood to thicken, increasing the workload for the heart while restricting the flow of blood throughout the entire body. Excess production of PAF is believed to be caused by modern lifestyle factors, including high stress, a diet high in processed (hydrogenated) fats, and chronic exposure to allergens. PAF also increases production of free radicals, promotes inflammation and increases formation of blood clots (thromboses) that are involved in heart disease, strokes, and peripheral vascular diseases, such as intermittent claudication. By inhibiting PAF, ginkgo improves circulation and helps to keep blood flowing freely. This enhances delivery of oxygen to the brain and central nervous system while reducing the risks of both clot formation and coronary arterial spasms that can lead to heart attacks.

Platelet-Activating Factor (PAF) *A compound that normally helps the body form clots to minimize blood loss from wounds.*

Ginkgo and High Blood Pressure

High blood pressure (hypertension) threatens an estimated 25 percent of Americans. Hypertension is associated with atherosclerosis, hypertensive renal failure, stroke, congestive heart failure, and myocardial infarction (heart attack). Japanese researchers showed that ginkgo extract was effective in significantly reducing blood pressure in hypertensive rats after twenty days of treatment. Additionally, the researchers noted that the rats did not show any increase in the size of their hearts, a known sign of sustained high blood pressure. Importantly, ginkgo normalizes high blood pressure only, with no effect on animals with normal blood pressure levels.

Ginkgo Protects Heart Tissues

Sudden cardiac tissue death is the leading cause of death in the United States, and occurs when the heart does not get enough oxygen and blood to properly contract and keep pumping blood to the rest of the body. Ginkgo has been shown to protect the heart by reducing blood pressure, reducing formation of blood clots, and increasing circulation to heart tissues. According to a study published in *Biochemistry and Biology International,* it also protects heart tissues from the acute damage caused by lack of oxygen after a heart attack, while helping the damaged tissues to heal from the effects of oxygen deprivation.

A large body of research shows that ginkgo can also prevent arrhythmia, a potentially fatal disruption of normal heart rhythm. In one experiment, after scientists induced heart attacks in rats, ginkgo actually protected the heart tissues from damage caused by a prolonged lack of oxygen for more than forty minutes. Moreover, it prevented the occurrence of arrhythmias that would normally be caused by the chemical and electrical imbalances present following a heart attack.

Ginkgo and Sexual Function

Male impotence is often due to poor circulation in the pelvic area. Since ginkgo increases the general circulation, it often helps to restore sexual function. In one study, ginkgo was found to be effective in improving erectile dysfunction in a group of impotent males taking 60 mg of ginkgo extract for six months. *The Journal of Urology* reported a second successful study involving sixty men who had previously failed to respond to Papaverine, an injectable prescription medication commonly used to treat male sexual dysfunction. Researchers suggested that ginkgo was working by stimulating the release of nitric oxide (NO), which signals the blood vessels to dilate to achieve and maintain an erection.

Ginkgo has also been shown to be an effective treatment for sexual problems related to the use of commonly prescribed antidepressant drugs, particularly the selective serotonin reuptake inhibitors (SSRIs). One group of thirty men and thirty-three women who were suffering from sexual side effects, ranging from decreased libido and erectile difficulties to delayed or inhibited orgasm, received ginkgo extract in doses ranging from 80 to 120 mg daily. After only four weeks, 84 percent of the patients reported positive results in all phases of the sexual response cycle. A major point of interest with this study is that women responded better than men, with 91 percent of women reporting improvements in the sexual response, as compared with 76 percent of the men.

Ginkgo and Vision and Hearing Problems

Age-related macular degeneration is among the leading causes of loss of vision. Ginkgo is believed to benefit this and other vision problems, such as glaucoma, cataracts, and diabetic retinopathy, by preventing free radical damage and by enhancing delivery of blood and oxygen to the retina to help repair tissues.

A systematic review of nineteen clinical studies found that ginkgo extract offered significant symptom reduction for tinnitus sufferers, particularly if treatment started soon after symptoms were first detected. In one double-blind study,

French researchers reported that when patients with tinnitus were treated with ginkgo extract, 40 percent reported marked relief from their symptoms, while others reported varying degrees of benefit.

Tinnitus
Internal "ringing" in the ears and similar noises perceived in the absence of any external noise.

Ginkgo has been shown to help control vertigo and dizziness, likely by promoting blood flow to aid the brain in accurately receiving and evaluating sensory information. When researchers treated seventy patients diagnosed with vertigo with 160 mg of ginkgo on a daily basis for three months, patients showed improvement in the intensity, frequency, and duration of vertigo symptoms. Improvements were noticed in as little as one month, and by the end of the study 47 percent of the ginkgo–extract-treated patients were completely free of vertigo symptoms. Based on the success of these studies, ginkgo extract should be taken at the first sign of problems with balance or vertigo.

Recommend Dosages

The typical dose of ginkgo is 40 to 80 mg three times daily of an extract of fifty parts alcohol to one part ginkgo standardized to contain 24-percent ginkgo-flavone glycosides. You may need to take supplements for six weeks before noticing results, so don't give up too soon. For some conditions, such as peripheral vascular disease, tinnitus, and dizziness, the recommended dose is higher—80 mg twice daily or 40 mg four times daily.

Safety and Cautions

Ginkgo is very safe. Extremely high doses have been given to animals without serious consequences. Ginkgo has shown no toxicity to the liver or kidneys and has not hampered new blood-cell formation. We still have no proof of its safety for pregnant and nursing women, however.

In all the clinical trials using ginkgo, involving a total of almost 10,000 patients, the incidence of side effects produced by ginkgo extract was extremely small, with just a few cases of nausea, heartburn, mild tension headache, dizziness, and allergic skin reactions. However, massive ginkgo overdoses have led to agitation, restlessness, and gastrointestinal distress.

According to the Commission E Monographs, German medical authorities do not believe that ginkgo interacts seriously with any drugs. However, because of ginkgo's blood-thinning effects, some authorities caution that it should not be combined with anticoagulants or even aspirin. There have been two case reports in highly regarded journals of subdural hematoma (bleeding in the skull) and hyphema (spontaneous bleeding into the iris chamber) in association with ginkgo use. Yet, if this risk is significant, it seems odd that similar side effects were not observed in the large number of patients who participated in the ginkgo clinical trials or have been using the herb for years in Germany.

CHAPTER 5

GINSENG AND ELEUTHERO— ENERGIZERS

In continuous use in China for more than 2,000 years, ginseng is called "the king of all tonics." It restores vital energy throughout the entire body, helping to overcome stress and fatigue. There are actually three different herbs commonly called ginseng: Asian ginseng (*Panax ginseng*), American ginseng (*Panax quinquefolius*), and Siberian ginseng (*Eleutherococcus senticosus*), which is not really ginseng at all but functions nearly identically. In fact, its labels are now required to read *Eleutherococcus senticosus* only.

Asian ginseng is a perennial that grows in northern China, Korea, and Russia. In traditional Chinese terms, Asian ginseng is seen as more *yang*, or stimulating. It raises body temperature, improves digestion, strengthens the lungs, and calms the spirit. Its close relative, American ginseng, is cultivated in the United States, though largely exported to Asia, where it is prized as a *yin* herb—less heating, less stimulating, and more balanced than Asian ginseng.

The active ingredients in ginseng are called ginsenosides. There are many different ones, each having its own specific effects. There have been two major reviews of ginseng research, surveying thirty-seven experiments done between 1968 and 1990, on a total of 2,562 cases, with treatments averaging two to three months. In thirteen studies, the individuals showed an improvement in mood, and in eleven, improvement in intellectual performance. All showed a near total absence of side effects.

Eleutherococcus senticosus grows primarily in China and Siberia. Russian scientists conducted the first modern research on this herb in the 1940s, concluding that eleuthero was as effective as Asian ginseng, with the added benefit of being substantially less expensive.

While each type of ginseng offers a unique set of properties, all increase resistance to stress, enhance mental alertness, and improve stamina and immunity. And all are referred to as *adaptogens.*

The Power of Adaptogens

Adaptogens are a group of remarkable substances that help the body adapt to stress from various sources, including extremes of temperature, radiation, and toxins. Adaptogens are also effective in helping the body cope with the stress of physical exertion, sleep deprivation, infections, and both physical and psychological trauma.

Respect for the benefits of adaptogens dates back thousands of years to ancient China, but serious scientific study didn't begin until the 1950s, when Soviet scientists thoroughly re searched adaptogens to help soldiers fight stress, reduce illness, build and maintain strong muscles, and enhance endurance. Adaptogens were found to be especially effective for helping the body return to a healthy state of balance (homeostasis) following periods of stress. For example, when blood pressure is too high, an adaptogen can lower it back to normal. Conversely, if blood pressure is too low, an adaptogen can raise it back to normal. Ginseng is often mistakenly called a stimulant, but it is actually a true adaptogen that works over time to support health.

Ancient Tonic for Modern Stress

Ginseng appears to protect us from stress, which is a significant health problem in modern-day life. Among its adaptogenic effects, ginseng also stimulates the mind, increases physical performance, strengthens immunity, and helps the hormones to better regulate bodily functions. It also helps to protect the liver, which might account for its ability to speed the processing of alcohol in the body. Ginseng also increases oxygen levels in the cells and tissues of the body to boost endurance, alertness, and visual-motor coordination. Its effect on brain function makes it useful for the elderly, and it combines well with ginkgo for maximum effect.

The ginsengs, especially eleuthero, support the adrenals, our stress-management glands. They provide the energy for the fight-or-flight response. When faced with a true emergency, this response can save your life. However, when we are overly stressed our adrenals continue to release adrenaline and cortisol, and in time, adrenal overstimulation can lead to exhaustion. A serious consequence of adrenal exhaustion is the sharp drop in our immune response, leaving us more vulnerable to colds, flu, and even more serious illnesses. It is estimated that at least 80 percent of visits to doctors are for stress-related illnesses, including heart disease, high blood pressure, and cancer. Thus, stress reduction must be a priority in our self-care.

Adrenal Glands
A pair of small, almond-shaped glands located on top of both kidneys that secrete steroid hormones, including cortisol, testosterone, and adrenaline, the "fight-or-flight" hormone.

Ginseng Enhances Immune Function

There is evidence of ginseng's ability to enhance immune function. In a double-blind placebo-controlled study, 227 people took either a 100 mg dose of ginseng or a placebo. After four weeks of supplementation, they were all given a flu vaccination. Those receiving the ginseng demonstrated lower incidence of colds and flus compared with the placebo group (15 cases versus 42). Researchers also discovered that antibody measurements in response to the vaccination were higher in the ginseng group.

Ginseng Improves Memory in Stroke Patients

Researchers in China have recently shown how ginseng protects and improves memory scores in patients following a stroke. Dementia, or memory loss, is frequently seen in the elderly—particularly following a stroke—and is a growing problem in aging populations around the world. Ginseng has been used in China for thousands of years to treat age-related diseases, but proof of its benefits following treatment for mild and moderate dementia in humans had not been reported previously.

The researchers randomly treated twenty-five stroke patients suffering from mild to moderate dementia with ginseng three times daily. Participants took memory tests measuring immediate and delayed story recall, delayed word recall, verbal learning, verbal recognition, and visual recognition at the beginning of the study and again after twelve weeks. Overall, the researchers reported that those patients receiving the ginseng showed significant improvement in their average memory scores after only twelve weeks of supplementation. Their study showed that ginseng effectively increases the activity of acetylcholine and choline acetyltransferase (ChAT), two important neurotransmitters (chemical messengers) involved in cognition and memory.

Ginseng Outperforms Drugs for Improving Post-Stroke Dementia

A second study demonstrated that ginseng was superior to a cognitive-enhancing drug in improving the memory of post-stroke dementia patients. Researchers studied forty patients (twenty-six men and fourteen women) who were diagnosed with mild to moderate dementia after suffering an ischemic (caused by lack of circulation) stroke. In a randomized, double-blind, controlled clinical trial, twenty-five subjects were given ginseng while fifteen subjects were treated with Duxil for twelve weeks. Duxil is a drug thought to increase oxygenation in brain tissues that is used to treat elderly dementia patients.

Dementia
Loss of brain function due to disease or trauma, which can include impaired decision making, judgment, memory spatial orientation, thinking, reasoning, and verbal communication.

The results of this study showed that the subjects treated with ginseng experienced greater benefits than the group taking the medication, with significant improvements in recalling stories and words, in verbal learning, and in verbal and visual recognition.

These results support the findings of previous animal studies that found that ginseng significantly improves learning and memory following transient cerebral ischemia, a type of stroke common in elderly patients wherein there is a brief incidence of reduced blood flow to a section of the brain, leading to lack of oxygen and resultant damage. As with the earlier study, ginseng was shown to help by increasing the activity of acetylcholine, a key brain neurotransmitter for learning and memory.

Additionally, ginseng can improve some aspects of mental function in healthy middle-aged men and women. In a two-month study of 112 people, subjects received either ginseng or a placebo. According to the researchers, those supplementing with ginseng showed improved abstract thinking ability.

Ginseng Improves Male Sexual Function

A recent study published in *The Journal of Urology* indicates that ginseng can improve sexual function in men with impotence. Korean researchers studied the effects of ginseng in forty-five men with erectile dysfunction in a randomized, crossover, double-blind study. The men took either 900 mg of ginseng or a placebo three times a day for eight weeks. After a two-week break, the treatments were switched for an additional eight-week period.

When the men were receiving ginseng, their scores for erectile function, sexual desire, and satisfaction during intercourse were higher compared with when they were taking the placebo. The men reported an increased ability to achieve and maintain an erection when on ginseng compared with when they were taking the placebo. In fact, 60 percent of the men said that their erections improved when they were on ginseng compared with only 20 percent when taking the placebo. The study's authors surmised that ginseng may improve erections by elevating the production of nitric oxide, a substance required for achieving and maintaining an erection.

Ginseng Is Beneficial for Diabetics

Because ginseng's adaptogenic effects help to lower blood pressure and enhance insulin production by the pancreas, it can be a useful adjunct in treating diabetes. In one study, ginseng was shown to help reduce blood glucose levels in diabetics. Researchers found that American ginseng (*Panax quinquefolius*) significantly lowered the blood sugar levels of diabetics taking part in a study conducted at the University of Toronto, Canada. Ten non-diabetic adults and nine adults with type II diabetes were given ginseng on four separate occasions, either forty minutes before a meal or during a meal, or given a placebo. Blood sugar levels were measured at fifteen and thirty-minute intervals for two hours after the meal. The researchers concluded that ginseng lowered the diabetics' blood sugar levels when compared with the placebo. Also, the researchers found it didn't matter if the ginseng was taken before or during the meal.

In similar studies, Korean ginseng (*Panax ginseng*) has also shown to stimulate insulin secretions in both diabetic and glucose-loaded normal test subjects, while nondiabetic subjects consuming a standard diet were not affected. In one double-blind study, thirty-six people with adult-onset diabetes received Korean ginseng at dosages of 100 mg or 200 mg daily. Those supplemented with ginseng showed improved blood sugar levels.

Ginseng has been shown to improve the ratio of LDL to HDL cholesterol, to aid in managing and treating heart disease and high blood pressure, and to help in all issues affecting diabetics, as well as others.

Ginseng and Endurance

Russian research shows how eleuthero can be used both for enhancing athletic purposes and for enhancing work capacity. It became popular with Russian Olympic teams, especially runners and weight lifters. Mountain climbers, sailors, and factory workers also were given Siberian ginseng, which enhanced their performance and reduced the number of days they were out sick. In one experiment, radio operators who took eleuthero daily for one month significantly increased their work capacity. In another study, skiers who took it prior to a race increased both their endurance and resistance to the effects of a cold.

Ginseng and Cancer Therapy

While ginseng is not, in and of itself, a cure or treatment for cancer, research shows that it helps people cope with the stress caused by cancer therapies. Ginseng has been shown to protect healthy cells from damage caused by radiation therapy. For example, in one study of eighty patients being treated for breast cancer, those receiving Siberian ginseng experienced less nausea and dizziness, and were better able to maintain a healthy appetite. Ginseng has also been shown to stimulate natural killer cells, the white blood cells that the body uses to attack cancer cells directly.

Safety and Dosages

Ginseng is available as a powdered root in capsules, as tablets, or as an alcohol-based tincture. The recommended dose of the more commonly used Asian ginseng is 100 to 200 mg daily of an extract standardized to contain 4- to 7-percent ginsenosides. The recommended dose for ginseng tincture is 5 ml twice daily of a concentration made of five parts alcohol to one part ginseng. Take ginseng for three weeks, and then take one week off.

Eleuthero should be taken at a dose of 200 to 400 mg daily of standardized extract containing more than 1-percent eleutherosides. Since it is less stimulating than Asian ginseng and has a milder effect on hormones, such as testosterone and estrogen, it can be taken for longer periods of time.

Side effects with ginseng are rare. However, as with any substance, allergy can occur. With Asian ginseng, menstrual abnormalities and breast tenderness have been reported. Overuse can cause overstimulation, including insomnia. There have also been unconfirmed reports of excessive doses raising the blood pressure and increasing the heart rate. In Chinese traditional medicine, ginseng is used during pregnancy, and there are no restrictions according to the Commission E Monographs either, although as with any herb, this should be done only under the care of a qualified healthcare practitioner.

CHAPTER 6

RHODIOLA ROSEA—
ADAPTOGEN

Another amazing adaptogen from the East with a long history of use is rhodiola (*rhodiola rosea*), also known as rose root, rose wort, golden root, and, because it grows in the cold Arctic regions of eastern Siberia, Arctic root. In addition to flourishing in cold climates, rhodiola has also adapted to very high altitudes—from 11,000 to 18,000 feet—producing yellow blossoms that smell like roses. Hence the Latin name, *rosea.*

Ancient folklore held rhodiola in special esteem for improving health and extending life. Three thousand years ago it was believed that those who drank rhodiola tea would live for more than 100 years, prompting ancient Chinese em - perors to dispatch expeditions to search for this potent herb. In Mongolia, rhodiola was used to treat cancer and tuberculosis, while in Georgia it was prescribed to fight fatigue, enhance endur - ance, and relieve depression. And in Siberia, rho- diola was traditionally given to newlyweds to enhance sexual potency, and improve chances of producing a healthy baby.

The Modern Science of Adaptogens
But this is not all just simple folklore. Modern sci- ence has confirmed that rhodiola has many impressive health benefits. Among these is its ability to improve concentration and physical

energy, balance stress hormones, restore healthy blood sugar and insulin levels in diabetics, and to improve mood and boost the immune system.

As an adaptogen, rhodiola appears to be at least as powerful as ginseng and protects against high levels of the stress hormone cortisol. However, it also stimulates both mental and physical performance. For this reason, it was extensively researched by the Soviet government and military scientists in the 1940s. This research was originally intended to improve the performance of Soviet soldiers on the battlefield and thus was a closely guarded state secret. Russian researchers were so impressed with rhodiola that it was given to Soviet athletes and later became a staple for cosmonauts to help them adapt to the stresses of returning to earth after long missions in space.

Rhodiola's Mental Effects

Rhodiola's effects on the brain are perhaps the most interesting. Numerous studies have shown that it helps to improve concentration and attention span, especially when one is tired. In one test, researchers found that during proofreading tests, subjects taking rhodiola decreased their number of errors by 88 percent! It works in part through its antioxidant function, protecting the brain against free radical damage, similar to the action of ginkgo.

Rhodiola has been shown to help the brain produce serotonin, an important neurotransmitter that helps to improve mood and maintain a sense of contentment. Russian researchers discovered that one of the ways rhodiola helps to relieve depression is by enhancing the transport of two important precursors, tryptophan and 5-hydroxytryptophan (5-HTP), in the brain to increase serotonin levels. In Russia, rhodiola is used to help treat seasonal affective disorder (SAD), a seasonal depressive illness seen in northern latitudes and caused by a lack of sunshine during long, dark winter months. In one study, 128 people suffering from depression were given 200 mg of rhodiola. Two-thirds of the patients experienced either a major reduction in the complete disappearance of all symptoms.

Serotonin
A neurotransmitter or brain chemical that promotes feelings of well-being, contentment, personal security, relaxation, confidence, and concentration.

Rhodiola and Heart Health

Rhodiola helps to control arrhythmias (erratic heartbeat). It has also been shown to restore cardiac health by reducing the release of adrenal hormones, such as catecholamines and corticosteroids, that are produced when the body is under stress. Left unchecked, these stress hormones elevate blood pressure and raise cholesterol levels. Rhodiola has been found to help prevent heart disease by reducing blood levels of cholesterol and other harmful fats that cause heart disease and promote hardening of the arteries.

Rhodiola and Cancer

Rhodiola also boosts the immune system, helping the body fight the formation and spread of cancer. As a potent antioxidant, rhodiola prevents damage to healthy cell membranes (lipid peroxidation) that is known to initiate many forms of cancer. Rhodiola also increases the production and enhances the activity of natural killer (NK) cells used by the immune system to destroy cancer cells. When researchers treated experimental animals, they discovered that rhodiola extract helped inhibit tumor growth by 39 per -

Natural Killer Cells
A type of lymphocyte (white blood cell) that attacks and destroys cancer cells and a wide variety of infectious agents by releasing a burst of chemicals that is lethal to invading organisms.

cent and reduced the spread of cancer cells (metastasis) by 50 percent.

Rhodiola was also found to aid in recovery from cancer by supporting the detoxifying function of the liver, which can be overwhelmed during traditional cancer therapies. It has been shown to be helpful in bladder cancer, and extracts have been shown to increase survival rates of several types of cancer, including adenocarcinoma and lung cancer.

Rhodiola and Fat Loss

On top of an already impressive list of benefits, rhodiola has also been shown to aid in weight control by helping to break down hard-to-lose stored body fat and to improve muscle-to-fat ratios. As anyone who has tried to lose weight quickly learns, losing stored fat is especially difficult. The key to breaking down and releasing stubborn stores of body fat is an important enzyme known as hormone-sensitive lipase (HSL). Hormone-sensitive lipase helps the body break

Enzymes
Biological substances (proteins) that act as catalysts to assist and promote countless complex cellular chemical reactions required for life.

down stored fats so that they are released and made available to be burned as energy. The key to stimulating hormone-sensitive lipase is the chemical known as cAMP (cyclic adenosine monophosphate). Research has shown that by helping to activate cAMP, rhodiola stimulates the release of hormone-sensitive lipase to facilitate the release of body fat, which is then burned as fuel for increased cellular energy.

When researchers treated volunteers with rhodiola extract, their serum levels of fatty acids went up 44 percent higher than those of untreated subjects after one hour of bicycle exercise. (Increased levels of fatty acids indicate that fat is being released from the cells.) And in another study, when rhodiola was combined with simply walking for thirty minutes, fat levels increased by 17 percent in the treated subjects. Lastly, when obese volunteers added rhodiola to their weight-loss program, they lost 11 percent of total body weight after only three months, compared with only 4 percent for untreated volunteers.

These impressive results show that rhodiola, combined with modest exercise and a sensible diet, can be a powerful aid in weight control by helping to activate fat burning enzymes to lose stubborn excess weight.

Choosing a Rhodiola Supplement

As with other herbs, make sure you are getting the real thing. There are many plant varieties of rhodiola, but the one that is known to be effective is called *Rhodiola rosea*. While it has many active ingredients, the key components are called rosavin and salidroside. So it is best to take rhodiola supplements that are standardized and can therefore guarantee at least 2 percent rosavin and 1 percent salidroside.

Suggested Dosage

Take 100 mg of standardized extract two to three times daily before meals.

Safety and Precautions

Rhodiola rosea is an extremely safe herb that is free of contraindications and side effects.

CHAPTER 7

TURMERIC— NATURE'S ANTI- INFLAMMATORY

Turmeric (*Curcuma longa*) is the pungent spice that gives curry its distinctive flavor and deep yellow color. Turmeric has been used since antiquity in hot, tropical regions such as India and southern Asia to keep foods fresh and prevent food poisoning. The ability to preserve foods is derived from turmeric's antioxidant and antimicrobial properties that help to prevent free radicals and bacterial pathogens from spoiling meats and other foods. But these antioxidant and antimicrobial benefits are not limited to food preservation. Turmeric has been used for 5,000 years in the ancient Indian medical tradition, Ayurveda, to preserve health by purifying the blood, protecting the liver, calming digestion, treating arthritis, and, applied externally, treating wounds and skin diseases.

Doctors are now using turmeric to treat certain cancers; inflammatory conditions, such as arthritis, osteoarthritis, inflammatory bowel syndrome, and psoriasis; and multiple sclerosis. Turmeric is also being studied for its efficacy in treating health conditions caused by free radical damage, such as cardiovascular disease, as well as for its role in protecting the liver from chemical injury.

The Power of Curcuminoids

Today we recognize that all of turmeric's health

benefits derive from a unique group of antioxidants called curcuminoids. These powerful compounds protect the body from oxidative damage from free radicals that causes various chronic conditions, including cardiovascular disease, cancer, neurological disorders, arthritis, and other aging-related degenerative diseases. In fact, curcuminoids are among the most potent of all known antioxidants, and are more than five times as potent as vitamin E (alpha-tocopherol) at reducing exceptionally dangerous free radicals, such as superoxide and peroxyl radicals.

Turmeric's Anti-inflammatory and Anti-arthritic Action

Turmeric is most well known for its powerful anti-inflammatory activity. Every day, millions of arthritis suffers turn to nonsteroidal anti-inflammatory drugs (NSAIDs), such as aspirin, ibuprofen, and naproxen, to alleviate the pain and inflammation of arthritis and osteoarthritis. NSAIDs help to reduce inflammation and pain by inhibiting prostaglandins, substances released in the body that promote inflammation. Unfortunately, while NSAIDs block production of "bad" (COX-2) prostaglandins responsible for inflammation, they also block "good" (COX-1) prostaglandins required to maintain and protect the lining of the stomach. Taken for too long, NSAIDs can cause gastrointestinal ulcerations and bleeding.

Inflammation
A defensive reaction that directs white blood cells and chemicals to attack bacteria and viruses.

When COX-2 inhibitors, such as celecoxib (Celebrex) and rofecoxib (Vioxx), were introduced they were considered to be superior to NSAIDs because of their ability to selectively inhibit only the inflammatory COX-2 enzymes to provide relief from pain and inflammation without the negative side effects. Unfortunately, even these drugs have been shown to cause serious side effects, including increasing blood pressure, fluid retention, and kidney failure. Now turmeric has been shown to be a safe and natural alternative to both NSAIDs and COX-2 inhibitors for controlling arthritis.

In Asia, extracts of turmeric have been used for centuries to treat inflammatory conditions such as arthritis. British researchers recently discovered that turmeric acts as a natural and potent COX-2 inhibitor, which may explain why so many people taking turmeric report experiencing relief from arthritis. In one clinical trial, persons suffering from rheumatoid arthritis reported significant relief from pain and inflammation following treatment with high doses of turmeric, up to 1,200 mg per day, with virtually no side effects.

Turmeric and Cancer Prevention

Following the introduction of COX-2 inhibitors, physicians began to notice that patients who took these drugs over several years were less likely than other patients to be diagnosed with colon cancer. These observations correlated with previous research that showed that COX-2 levels are abnormally high in certain cancers.

Now researchers have found that inflammatory COX-2 enzymes are involved in a number of cancers, including cancer of the colon and pancreas. Researchers have found that turmeric extract significantly inhibits the growth rate of human pancreatic cancer cells in test tube experiments.

Curcumin, the active ingredient that gives turmeric its bright yellow color, has also proven effective in fighting prostate cancer cells. Researchers have discovered that when curcumin is combined with a naturally occurring molecule called TRAIL (tumor necrosis factor-related apoptosis-inducing ligand), the two agents killed two to three times more cancer cells than either treatment by itself. The combination killed up to 80 percent of the cancer cells.

Curcumin has also been shown to stop the spread of multiple myeloma, a cancer of the bone marrow. Researchers from the MD Anderson Cancer Center at the University of Texas discovered that turmeric extract stopped the activation of processes involved in the spreading of myeloma cells. Curcumin was also shown to trigger apoptosis, a process that causes cells to commit suicide, in the cancer cells. Based on the results of their study, the researchers suggested that patients suffering from multiple myelomas be treated with this "pharmacologically safe agent."

Apoptosis
A controlled biological process that causes a cell to self-destruct. This form of "cellular suicide" is a natural phenomenon that plays an important role in maintaining healthy tissues.

Turmeric Prevents Alzheimer's Disease

Interest in turmeric's ability to protect brain tissues was stimulated by studies that revealed very low levels of neurological diseases such as Alzheimer's in elderly Indian populations. Other researchers had noted that, in addition to reducing the incidence of certain cancers, people routinely taking COX-2 medications for years have a lower incidence of Alzheimer's disease (AD).

Suspecting that inflammation played a role in Alzheimer's disease led scientists to the discovery that COX-2 plays a role in the formation of the plaques found in the brains of people diagnosed with AD. Yet despite the obvious potential benefits of using COX-2 inhibitors to prevent

Alzheimer's disease, physicians have avoided making such recommendations because of the serious side effects associated with the drugs.

Looking for a safer alternative to the COX-2 inhibitors, researchers turned to animal studies with turmeric, which has been shown effective for suppressing COX-2 without any side effects. They found that turmeric was effective, offering a safe alternative to protect against the ravages of Alzheimer's disease. This benefit was further confirmed when researchers at the University of California, Los Angeles, reported that turmeric appeared to slow the progression of Alzheimer's in mice.

Turmeric and Heart Disease

Turmeric has been found to support heart health in a number of ways. First, it has been shown to lower blood cholesterol levels. In one study, healthy humans taking 500 mg of turmeric per day for seven days had a 29 percent reduction in serum cholesterol levels. Additionally, test subjects had a 33 percent drop in blood lipid peroxides known to damage arteries and contribute to heart disease. The authors of this study stated that they felt these results were indicative of a potential role of curcuminoids as a heart disease preventative.

Turmeric Lowers Fibrinogen

Turmeric also helps to prevent the formation of dangerous blood clots that can lead to heart attack. Elevated blood levels of fibrinogen, a protein used to form blood clots, are now recognized as a major risk factor for coronary heart disease (heart attacks) and cerebrovascular disease (strokes). These together account for about 60 percent of deaths in the elderly. In fact, many researchers now consider fibrinogen levels to be a greater predictor for heart disease and strokes than cholesterol or homocysteine levels. Additionally high fibrinogen levels have also been associated with a number of other diseases, including cancer, diabetes, and hypertension. Unfortunately, fibrinogen levels are known to rise with age, and there are no pharmaceutical drugs available for lowering fibrinogen.

When researchers treated subjects with elevated fibrinogen levels with 20 mg of turmeric extract per day, levels plummeted after only fifteen days of treatment. No adverse effects were noted by any of the subjects, nor were there any adverse changes in any other blood chemistries.

Turmeric and Multiple Sclerosis

New animal research suggests that turmeric may play a role in blocking the progression of multiple sclerosis (MS). In multiple sclerosis, the body's immune system attacks the protective myelin sheath surrounding nerve fibers in the brain and spine. Symptoms of multiple sclerosis include muscle weakness and stiffness, balance and coordination problems, numbness and vision disturbances.

Researchers treated groups of mice bred with autoimmune encephalomyelitis (EAE)—an auto - immune condition similar to multiple sclerosis— with turmeric in varying doses. Then, they monitored the mice for signs of MS-like neurological impairment and compared them with a control. After fifteen days, mice that had not been treated with turmeric suffered from complete paralysis of both hind limbs. In contrast, mice treated with turmeric showed only minor symptoms, such as a temporarily stiff tail. And mice receiving the highest doses of turmeric remained completely unimpaired throughout the full thirty days of the study.

And as with the previously mentioned low rate of Alzheimer's disease in India, researchers again noted that in other Asian countries, such as China, where turmeric consumption is high, there are very few reports of MS.

Suggested Dosage

Take 100 mg of standardized extract two to three times daily before meals.

Safety and Precautions

Turmeric is extremely safe, with some people regularly consuming as much as 4 grams daily without adverse effects. Due to its ability to lower blood-clotting factors, such as fibrinogen, people taking anticoagulant medications should consult with a doctor prior to taking large doses of turmeric.

CHAPTER 8

MILK THISTLE—
LIVER SUPPORTER

The seeds, fruit, and leaves of milk thistle (*Silybum marianum*) have been used for medicinal purposes for more than 2,000 years. The Roman writer Pliny the Elder, who lived from A.D. 23 to 79, reported that the juice of milk thistle mixed with honey "could carry off bile." In Europe, the herb was used widely up through the early twentieth century for the treatment of liver ailments as well as insufficient lactation. The active ingredients in milk thistle appear to be four substances known collectively as silymarin, of which the most potent is silibinin. When injected intravenously, silibinin is one of the few known antidotes to poisoning by the deathcap mushroom, *Amanita phalloides*.

Silymarin is a powerful antioxidant. We are constantly exposed to toxins such as cigarette smoke, car exhaust, pesticides, and other chemicals in our air, food, and water. This is in addition to the toxins that our bodies produce as by-products of our own metabolism. All these toxins produce free radicals, which cause cell damage. They can, however, be neutralized by substances called antioxidants. Two major antioxidants produced by the body, glutathione and superoxide dismutase (SOD), are greatly enhanced by silymarin. Thus, milk thistle acts as an antioxidant in the liver, protecting it from free-radical damage. Animal studies suggest that milk thistle extract can also protect against many poisons, from toluene, a common solvent, to acetaminophen, the main ingredient in Tylenol.

In Europe, doctors often prescribe milk thistle as extra protection for patients taking medications that are known to cause liver problems. I often recommend it to patients who are on medications such as antidepressants, which are metabolized (broken down) in the liver. Milk thistle can also protect against toxic exposure.

Milk Thistle and Liver Disease

Jaundice
A serious health condition caused by stress or damage to the liver that results in the skin and the whites of the eyes turning yel- low from deposits of excess bile.

The main constituent of milk thistle seeds, silymarin, is used to treat liver disease. Silymarin protects the cells against toxins and stimulates new cell growth in the liver. Based on the extensive folk use of milk thistle in cases of jaundice, European medical researchers have done serious research on the herb's medicinal effects. Milk thistle is widely used to treat alcoholic hepatitis, alcoholic fatty liver, liver cirrhosis, liver poisoning, and viral hepatitis. Milk thistle is one of the few herbs that has no equivalent in the drug world, with only two other natural substances, alpha-lipoic acid and N-acetylcysteine, having similar effects.

Treatment with milk thistle often produces significant improvement in, and relief from, common symptoms of chronic liver disease, including nausea, weakness, loss of appetite, fatigue, and pain. The blood levels of the liver enzymes, which are elevated in liver disease or damage, frequently go down.

Milk Thistle and Cirrhosis

Alcohol consumption and alcoholism take a

heavy toll on the liver, which is the chemical factory of the body. It is here that alcohol is broken down into its metabolites. Silymarin is useful for preserving the liver, although research shows that abstinence is the best treatment. One study observed 106 Finnish soldiers with mild alcoholic liver disease. The group treated with milk thistle had a significant improvement in liver function as measured by blood tests and a biopsy. (In a biopsy, a small piece of liver tissue is examined under a microscope.) Other studies have shown similar results. Again, however, research shows that abstinence from alcohol is still a better treatment than milk thistle.

Two different long-term controlled studies showed how milk thistle prolonged the life of patients with liver cirrhosis. In one study, 170 patients were given either milk thistle or a placebo and were observed for three to six years. After four years, 58 percent of the milk-thistle group had survived, compared with only 38 percent of the placebo group. Double-blind studies of patients with chronic viral hepatitis have shown that milk thistle can produce marked improvement in symptoms such as fatigue, reduced appetite, and abdominal discomfort, as well as in the levels of the liver enzymes.

Milk Thistle and Hepatitis

Hepatitis is a growing health problem that causes serious inflammation of the liver. The most common types of hepatitis viruses are A, B, and C, of which hepatitis A virus is the least serious type. Hepatitis B currently afflicts more than a million people, and hepatitis C has reached epidemic proportions, infect-

Hepatitis
Serious inflammation of the liver, generally viral in origin, the most common being hepa-titis C, which is a leading cause of liver cancer.

ing 4 million people in the United States alone—that's four times the number of people infected with HIV. Hepatitis C is responsible for some 10,000 deaths each year, and this rate is expected to triple by the end of the decade. Hepatitis C is also the most common cause of chronic liver diseases, such as cirrhosis, and is a leading cause of liver cancer.

Interferon (INF) and ribavarin, the current standard of medical treatment for hepatitis C, are effective for less than 30 percent of all patients after a year of treatment. And of those patients who do benefit from interferon, up to 70 percent of patients suffer a relapse within a few months of treatment. In total, only about 10 to 15 percent of hepatitis C patients enjoy a sustained recovery lasting even six months following treatment with interferon, and a slightly higher number of patients benefit from treatment with pegylated interferon.

While conventional treatments are not very successful against hepatitis, silymarin, especially when combined with other beneficial nutrients, is an excellent treatment. A patient of mine, a fifty-year-old man with elevated liver enzymes due to an old case of hepatitis, responded well to milk thistle treatment. His elevated enzymes came down to normal after eight weeks, and his symptoms of depression, fatigue, and nausea cleared as well.

Dosage Recommendations

The standard dosage of milk thistle is 200 mg two to three times a day of an extract standardized to contain 70-percent silymarin complex. There is some evidence that silymarin bound to the nutrient phosphatidylcholine is better ab - sorbed. This combination supplement should be taken at a dose of 100 to 200 mg twice a day.

Medical supervision is essential in all cases of liver disease, since liver disease is a very serious condition.

Safety and Precautions

Milk thistle and its silymarin extract are basically nontoxic, causing only the mildest of side effects in a small minority of patients. A study involving 2,637 patients showed a low incidence of side effects, limited primarily to mild gastrointestinal distress. Milk thistle is safe for use by pregnant and nursing mothers. Researchers have even felt safe enough to enroll pregnant women in the studies on silymarin.

CHAPTER 9

ST. JOHN'S WORT—
MOOD STABILIZER

St. John's wort (*Hypericum perforatum*) is a bushy perennial plant with yellow flowers that grows wild in many parts of the world, including Europe, Asia, and the United States. It gets its unusual name from St. John the Baptist, since it was traditionally collected on St. John's Day, June 24th. "Wort" is the Old English word for "plant." St. John's wort provides all the benefits of prescription antidepressants without any of the side effects, and at one-tenth the cost. By the year 2000, St. John's wort was one of the top-selling natural treatments for mild to moderate depression.

Like most medicinal plants, St. John's wort contains a complex mix of more than two dozen known active ingredients, each with its own unique effects. Together, these compounds synergize to provide greater health benefits than any one ingredient can offer on its own. This translates to greater healing power without any of the unwanted side effects found in many drugs composed of single, isolated compounds or synthetic chemicals. One ingredient, hypericin, while not the main antidepressant, is used as the marker for standardization of St. John's wort products. However, research by Professor W.E. Muller at the University of Frankfurt suggests that hyperforin may be the main antidepressant component.

Initially thought to be an inhibitor of MAO, an enzyme that breaks down neurotransmitters, St. John's wort more likely acts to increase the availability of the antidepressant neuro-transmitters, including sero-tonin, norepinephrine, and dopamine. It, therefore, is similar in action to the vari-ous antidepressant drugs.

Neurotransmitters
Chemical messengers in the brain, of which serotonin, norepinephrine, and dopamine are the best known. Deficiencies can produce depression.

In my own practice, and in the many communications I have received from now-happy users of St. John's wort, I have to conclude that, while it may not be the "magic bullet" for everyone, it certainly has a significant role in the treatment of depression. Many report feeling relieved of their depression, and, for those who had taken pharmaceutical antidepressants, it came without the familiar mood-dulling or "chemical" effects.

St. John's Wort and Depression

Researchers have shown that St. John's wort is effective for treating patients with depression, helping to relieve a wide range of symptoms, including sadness, helplessness, hopelessness, anxiety, headache, and exhaustion. And it does all this with minimal side effects.

In 1996, a significant and extensive review article on St. John's wort was published in the respected *British Medical Journal*. The authors did a meta-analysis, or summary and comparison, of twenty-three randomized clinical trials to look for overall conclusions. Fifteen studies compared the herb with a placebo, and eight compared it with conventional antidepressants, in a total of 1,757 outpatients. The research showed that St. John's wort worked nearly three times better than the placebos, with a success rate of

55 percent, versus only 22 percent in the placebo groups.

The meta-analysis just mentioned also compared the herb with a number of antidepressant drugs, and showed that St. John's wort worked slightly better, eliciting a positive response 64 percent of the time versus 59 percent for the antidepressants. In addition, only 0.8 percent of the people taking the herb dropped out of the study because of side effects, whereas 3 percent of those on the drug treatment dropped out.

Anyone with the symptoms of depression should get a thorough medical examination to rule out other possible causes of the symptoms. Medical conditions such as thyroid disorders, anemia, hypoglycemia, chronic fatigue syndrome, and nutritional deficiencies can also cause depression. More severe depression may also be unresponsive and, consequently, require stronger medication.

Controversial Study on Major Depression

One clinical study, published in the *Journal of the American Medical Association* (*JAMA*) in 2002, concluded that St. John's wort was not effective in treating depression, and the media reported it as such. What they failed to mention was that the population studied was suffering from severe depression, and that the prescription antidepressant, sertraline (Zoloft), with which it was compared, fared no better! The fact is, St. John's wort has been a well-validated treatment for mild to moderate depression in at least thirty studies on more than 1,700 patients. Thus, for those taking or considering taking St. John's wort for mild to moderate depression, it is still an excellent choice. Medication may be required in some cases, but it is over-prescribed, considering the success of natural medicines such as St. John's wort for "the blues," without the side effects of headache, lack of libido, nausea, withdrawal effects, and many others.

St. John's Wort and Seasonal Affective Disorder (SAD)

St. John's wort has been quite successful in the treatment of seasonal affective disorder (SAD), a condition brought on by the lack of sunlight that occurs in autumn and winter. SAD is especially common in countries at extreme northern and southern latitudes, where there are fewer sunlight hours during the winter months. The reduced hours of light trigger complex biochemical changes in the brain that cause symptoms such as depression, impaired concentration, anxiety, marked decrease in energy and libido, and carbohydrate cravings. Yet, when affected individuals get their required doses of sunlight, they feel energetic and ready to get on with their lives. In a study comparing St. John's wort to light therapy, the researchers concluded that St. John's wort is as effective as light therapy. This herb, they wrote, "brings light into dark places."

St. John's Wort and Sleep

St. John's wort works with the body's own sleep-promoting mechanism, the release of melatonin, to bring on restful sleep, without the hangover or addictive effects of prescription sedatives. One study showed that a dose of ninety drops a day over a three-week period significantly increased the nighttime melatonin level. Since it can take about a

Melatonin

A hormone secreted by the pineal gland to regulate the sleep-wake cycles in response to changes in light levels. At night, the lack of light triggers the release of melatonin to induce sleep.

week for this effect to begin, St. John's wort is recommended mainly for recurring insomnia, not for just the occasional restless night.

While St. John's wort won't take stress away, it will help you deal with it more easily. Since it needs to build up in the system to be most effective, you must take it regularly, at the usual dose, and not just before stressful events,

St. John's Wort and PMS

PMS is a common complaint that occurs in many women about seven days prior to the onset of their period, with moodiness, irritability, bloating, and fatigue. Many women report that their PMS and menstrual cramps, or menopausal symptoms, stopped after they began taking St. John's wort for depression. Some women begin taking it just before the onset of PMS. Others find that the herb needs time to build up in the system, so they take it all month long, with extra doses as needed.

Dosage and Safety

St. John's wort has been used safely, with no ill effects, by many depressed patients in Europe for years. There are generally no withdrawal effects from St. John's wort, so you can stop and restart as needed. After a few months, it's a good idea to assess if you still need St. John's wort and at what dosage. To do this, taper your dosage gradually, as opposed to stopping all at once.

The standard dose of St. John's wort is 300 mg three times a day of an extract standardized to contain 0.3-percent hypericin. Alternately, some people take 450 mg twice a day, or 600 mg in the morning and 300 mg in the evening. If stomach upset occurs, take it with food. For some, St. John's wort can be stimulating and thus should be avoided close to bedtime. Most report that it helps them to fall asleep more easily.

Many of my patients report positive effects almost immediately, with a sensation of "a weight being lifted," decreased anxiety, and an enhanced ability to concentrate. As with most antidepressants, though, it may take three or four weeks before you notice a significant effect.

St. John's wort can also be combined with adaptogens that can help to boost the positive effects.

Combining St. John's Wort with Other Antidepressants

St. John's wort should not be combined with an MAO inhibitor. Also, when combining agents that act on serotonin, there is a risk of serotonin syndrome—a cluster of symptoms that occurs as a result of elevated serotonin levels. Thus, medical supervision is essential if you are combining St. John's wort with an SSRI (such as Prozac, Zoloft, and Celexa).

Be alert for the signs of serotonin syndrome. While rare, this condition has the following symptoms: a dangerous rise in blood pressure, diarrhea, fever, severe anxiety, headache, muscle tension, and confusion. The first sign is often a severe, throbbing headache. If this occurs, immediately stop both the herb and the medication, and report to your physician. Psychiatrists have been successful in helping people transition well from medication to St. John's wort, using them in combination during the transition.

Switching from Other Antidepressants to St. John's Wort

Changing from an MAO-inhibiting antidepressant drug to St. John's wort requires a four-week "washout" period between stopping the drug and starting the herb to avoid a dangerous rise in blood pressure.

In switching from other types of antidepressants to St. John's wort, the two can often be combined, with a gradual reduction of medication and a gradual increase in the St. John's wort dose. Over a period of several weeks, the medication is phased out, and you are now on a full dose of the herb. **This must be done under a doctor's supervision.**

Side Effects and Cautions

St. John's wort is essentially free of side effects, with infrequent occurrence of mild stomach discomfort, allergic rashes, fatigue, or restlessness. Excessive sensitivity to sunlight can occur in fair-skinned individuals taking higher doses, so proper precautions should be taken. Older reports suggested that St. John's wort works like the class of drugs known as MAO inhibitors, leading to restrictions such as avoiding aged cheese, red wine, and decongestants. However, this concern is no longer considered valid. Although there is no evidence of its causing fetal damage or harm to nursing infants, St. John's wort has not been approved for use during pregnancy or while nursing.

Herb-Drug and Herb-Nutrient Interactions

It has been reported that St. John's wort interferes with the efficacy of a number of medications, by either decreasing or increasing their levels in the body. It should not be taken in combination with protease inhibitors (used in HIV and AIDS), cyclosporin (taken after organ transplants), digoxin, warfarin (Coumadin), and possibly, oral contraceptives. For some perspective, it turns out that grapefruit juice has similar effects in combination with many drugs, so one must be vigilant of food-drug interactions, as well.

Some clients occasionally take St. John's wort along with 5-hydroxytryptophan (5-HTP), a popular supplement that many people take for relief from depression, PMS, insomnia and obsessive-compulsive disorders. Both St. John's wort and 5-HTP increase the level of serotonin and can complement each other. While the possibility is theoretical, with no reported cases, it is advisable to watch for signs of too much serotonin, as described on page 65.

CHAPTER 10

SAW PALMETTO— PROMOTER OF PROSTATE HEALTH

Saw palmetto (*Serenoa repens*) is an extract of the saw palmetto berry, the fruit of a short palm tree that grows in the southeastern United States, mainly in Florida and Georgia. Native Americans traditionally used saw palmetto ber - ries to treat various urinary problems in men, as well as for breast disorders in women. European and American physicians at one time used the herb extensively as a treatment for benign prostatic hypertrophy (BPH), but in the United States, its use, as with all healing herbs, declined with the introduction of modern pharmaceuticals and drug patents.

Modern-day interest in saw palmetto was re-ignited in the 1960s, when French scientists conducted new research that ultimately led to the development of modern extracts. Interest in saw palmetto surged and today it is the main treatment for BPH and chronic prostatitis, or inflammation of the prostate, in both Europe and the United States.

Benign Prostatic Hypertrophy

Benign prostatic hypertrophy, or BPH, is a benign (noncancerous) enlargement of the prostate gland, affecting at least 10 percent of men by age forty and 50 percent of men by age fifty.

The prostate gland is involved in the production of seminal fluid. More important , though, is that this gland, which is the size of a walnut, sur-rounds the urethra, the tube through which the urine flows from the bladder. As the prostate enlarges, it narrows the urethral passageway, im-pairing the flow of the urine and causing a host of other problems. The typical symptoms of BPH include trouble starting urination, straining upon urination, a weak urinary stream, frequent urina-tion, dribbling after urination, a sensation of incom-plete emptying, and waking up several times at night to urinate. More serious problems include repeated bladder infections, involuntary urina-tion, and bleeding.

Treating BPH is big business. The prescription drugs Proscar (finasteride) and Hytrin (terazosin) are the standard medical choices for treatment. They are also very expensive, with a year's supply of Proscar costing about $800. By comparison, treatment with saw palmetto costs just a fraction of that.

The old treatment was surgery, specifically transurethral resection of the prostate (TURP). In this surgery, the excess prostate tissue surround-ing the urethra is cut away, enlarging the urethral opening, sort of like Roto-Rooter for the urethra. While the drugs are an improvement over this painful procedure, the herb is better yet.

Saw Palmetto Benefits BPH

The male hormone testosterone is changed in the prostate to a more active form called dihy-drotestosterone (DHT), which is a major cause of BPH. Saw palmetto works in two ways. It blocks 5-alpha-reductase, the enzyme that causes this change, and further blocks the binding of DHT to any cells. In addition to causing benign prostatic hypertrophy, DHT (dihydrotestosterone) also attacks hair follicles, cutting off the blood supply and leading to thinning and balding (alopecia).

There have been many double-blind studies comparing the benefits of saw palmetto with a placebo, with excellent results. One typical month-long study involved 110 patients taking 320 mg of saw palmetto daily. There was a significant increase in urinary flow and a decrease in nighttime urination.

About 90 percent of men respond to saw palmetto to some extent, beginning after approximately four to six weeks of treatment. Furthermore, while the prostate tends to continue growing when left untreated, saw palmetto causes a small but definite shrinkage. In other words, the herb does not simply relieve the symptoms, but may actually arrest the prostate enlargement.

Saw palmetto is often combined with other herbs, including nettles (*Urtica dioica*) and pygeum (*Pygeum africanum*). A German study of 2,080 patients combined saw palmetto with nettles over a twelve-week period, with a significant improvement in symptoms. The subjects were given 160 mg of saw palmetto and 120 mg of nettles twice daily. In another study, 250 men used either 50 mg of pygeum twice daily or a placebo along with the saw palmetto. The pygeum group did twice as well, with 66 percent showing improve - ment as compared with 33 percent of the pla - cebo group.

As Effective as Proscar, without Side Effects

A recent double-blind study followed 1,098 men who took either saw palmetto or Proscar (finasteride) for six months. The treatments were equally effective, but while the Proscar caused impotence in some of the men, the saw palmetto caused no significant side effects. Proscar also lowers the blood levels of prostatic specific antigen (PSA), which rises in prostate cancer, so its use may have the unintended effect of masking prostate cancer. Saw palmetto, on the other hand, leaves the PSA level unchanged, making it safer in this regard. Other studies have shown that saw palmetto is about as effective as the drugs alfuzosin (Uroxatral) and terazosin (Hytrin), minus their side effects—or prices.

Saw Palmetto and Women

There are a number of conditions in women, including some types of acne, excessive hair growth (hirsutism), and fibrocystic breasts, which are the result of increased male-hormone production. Saw palmetto has the same action in women as it does in men of lowering the DHT level.

Dosage and Safety

The standard dose of saw palmetto is 160 mg twice a day of an extract standardized to contain 85 to 95 percent fatty acids and sterols, which are the active ingredients in the herb. A once-a-day dose of 320 mg may work just as well. The recommended dose of saw palmetto tincture is 2 to 5 ml three times daily of a concentration of one part herb to five parts alcohol.

The side effect of saw palmetto, which is rare, is usually mild digestive disturbance. Proscar, on the other hand, can cause impotence, decreased libido, and impaired sexual functioning. Saw palmetto, meanwhile, actually improves sexual function. Which would you prefer?

CHAPTER 11

HOW TO
BUY AND USE
HERBAL MEDICINES

Selecting an herbal product—a tablet, capsule, tincture, or raw herb—can be confusing. Not only do different brands stress various features and benefits, but one often hears stories about ineffective products, leaving the consumer feeling helpless in sorting out all the information. In this chapter, you will learn about the different forms in which herbal medicines are sold and how to shop for quality products.

Herbs can be purchased as teas, tinctures, tablets, and capsules. Teas and tinctures, as liquids, are absorbed more rapidly than the other forms. In addition, traditional herbalists often recommend the liquid form because, in tasting the herb, we begin the process of allowing it to heal us. Tablets and capsules are made from measured amounts of an herb, and are the most common and convenient forms. Gelatin or vegetable-based capsules filled with powdered dried herb come in a variety of sizes and strengths, so you need to read the labels to ensure the proper dose. Tablets are powdered herb compressed into a solid pill, often with a variety of inert ingredients as fillers. They take longer to break down and be absorbed, and sometimes, depending on quality, may pass completely through the digestive system completely intact!

The whole herb, found in dried form in dark-colored glass jars at specialty herb shops, can be made into varying concentrations of teas in the form of *decoctions* (the strongest) or *infusions*. Chinese medicine often uses decoctions, made by boiling a combination of dried herbs for a while to extract the medicine and reduce the liquid, thereby concentrating the tea. A weaker tea is called an infusion, and is made the way we usually make tea from tea leaves or tea bags. Pour boiling water over the herb, let it steep, strain the liquid (or remove the tea bag), and then drink the mixture. The common soothing herb chamomile is often prepared this way.

A *tincture* is made by soaking the selected herb in alcohol. Some tinctures are made with glycerin to avoid the alcohol taste, but the resulting extract is weaker. If you prefer not to ingest alcohol, put the tincture in warm water or tea for a few minutes and let the alcohol evaporate, which also serves to disguise any remnant of the alcohol taste.

Check Labels Carefully

The first thing to look for is the common name of the herb—for example, St. John's wort—followed by the Latin botanical name, in this case, *Hypericum perforatum,* to be sure that you are getting the right plant source. This can be confusing at times, especially when manufacturers attempt to substitute an inactive relative for the proper herb, such as *Rhodiola sacra* instead of *Rhodiola rosea*, which contains the active ingredient rosavin. Next, look for the amount of herb in each unit—that is, capsule, tablet, or dropper—in grams (g or gm) or milligrams (mg). If the product is an extract, which is a concentrated form, the label should show the percent of the constituent to which the herb is standardized—for example, 0.3 percent hypericin for St. John's wort, and 24 percent ginkgolides for ginkgo.

Standardized Extracts

Unlike synthetic drugs, which are often a single compound, herbs frequently contain a variety of active ingredients. And since plants grow rather than being manufactured, the actual amount of a given active ingredient can be affected by a number of variables—where the plant was grown, when it was grown, the season in which it was harvested, and even the time of day it was harvested.

Marker
A compound used as a convenient reference point when creating standardized extracts to ensure that you get a specific amount of activity from each dosage unit.

Reputable manufacturers will make standardized herbal extracts that accommodate for these variations. They ensure a dependable product that delivers a consistent, measured amount of product per unit dose, be it a capsule, tablet, or tincture.

When making a standardized extract, manufacturers choose one ingredient, usually the one considered to be the active ingredient, as the reference point, or marker.

Even when the compound turns out not to be the active ingredient, it is often kept as the marker for convenience. For example, hypericin was initially considered to be the main active antidepressant ingredient in St. John's wort. Later research revealed that hypericin may not be as significant in this regard as hyperforin, yet the hypericin content has continued to be used as the marker for standardized extracts. Still other ingredients may also be involved in the herb's antidepressant action, and they are probably distributed within the plant in a way similar to that of hypericin. As a result, the hypericin standardization serves as a useful guidepost for the strength of all of the active ingredients in a St. John's wort product.

Simply taking an isolated "active compound" does not do justice to the power of the combination found in nature. They work synergistically for maximum effect. Moreover, traditional Chinese medicine almost always administers herbs in mixtures to utilize the synergistic properties of the various herbs.

Choosing the Correct Dose

All labels of herbal products provide dosage recommendations. Often the stated dosage is an average dose. A ginkgo label, for example, might suggest taking one 60-mg tablet, twice daily. This is meant to be a guideline, based on research and clinical use. While such a dose might improve memory, twice that dose is needed to treat Alzheimer's disease. We are all different and have varying requirements, so the dose ought to be individualized by careful experimentation and observation.

Generally, I recommend that people start with a relatively low dose, watch for a response—including potentially unwanted effects—and adjust the dose accordingly. I have had patients who did well taking 300 mg of St. John's wort once a day, while others needed four times that dose. Most fall in the middle, with the recommended 300 mg three times daily of a 0.3 percent hypericin extract.

The Truth about Labels

Herbal labels don't print much in the way of useful information, such as telling you what the herb should be used for. The reason for this seemingly deliberate lack of vital information is that most herbal products are regulated as dietary supplements. In 1994, the FDA's Dietary Supplement Health and Education Act (DSHEA) set new guidelines regarding the quality, labeling, packaging, and marketing of supplements. DSHEA allows manufacturers to make "statements of nutritional support for conventional vitamins and minerals," but since herbs aren't nutritional in the conventional sense, DSHEA allows them to make only what they call "structure and function claims." This means that a label can explain how a vitamin or herb affects the structure or function of the body. However, it can make no therapeutic or prevention claims, such as, "treats headaches," or, "cures the common cold." A saw palmetto label can say, "helps maintain urinary and prostate health in men fifty and over." But it cannot say, "treats benign prostatic hypertrophy," despite that being the reason for using it.

CONCLUSION

Herbal medicines are effective and safe natural remedies. They generally have fewer side effects than drugs and are also relatively inexpensive. They are anything but unproven folklore. Scientific studies have provided a wealth of information about how they work, all to our benefit.

If you've read this book from cover to cover, you now have a basic understanding of how some of the most popular medicinal herbs work and how to select them for your own use. They are nature's gift, working with our own bodies' chemistry and energy to promote healing and optimal health. They can hold their own against pharmaceuticals, and even do many things that pharmaceuticals cannot.

Since our natural resources are dwindling, it's important to remember that with the widening use of herbs, we must be sure to replant and renew. There is no sense in using these miraculous products to promote our own health while threatening the health of the planet. Moreover, any damage we do to nature comes right back to haunt us. As we destroy the rainforests, for example, we compromise our oxygen supply, literally choking ourselves in the process. We also are irrevocably losing hundreds of medicinal plants daily in this destruction.

My final words are a reminder to honor your mother, the Earth, and to walk lightly on her surface.

REFERENCES

Alder R, Lookinland S, Berry JA, Williams M. A Systematic Review of the Effectiveness of Garlic as an Anti-hyperlipidemic Agent. *Journal of the American Academy of Nurse Practitioners,* 2003; 15(3):120–129.

Press Release: "Ginkgo biloba for Alzheimer's Disease—'Promising Evidence'," October 21, 2002. Alzheimer's Society Dementia Care and Re - search. (www.alzheimers.org.uk/news_events/Press Release/m_ 021021Ginkgo.htm)

Birks J, Grimley Evans J, Van Dongen M. *Ginkgo Biloba* for Cognitive Impairment and Dementia (Cochrane Review). from: *The Cochrane Library, Issue 4, 2003.* Chester, UK: Wiley & Sons, Ltd.

Braeckman J. The Extract of *Serenoa Repens* in the Treatment of Benign Prostatic Hyperplasia: A Multicenter Open Study. *Current Therapeutic Research,* 1994; 55:776–785.

Braunig B, et al. Echinacea Purpurea Radix for Strengthening the Immune Response in Flu-Like Infections. *Zeitschrift fur Phytotherapie,* 1992; 13:7–13.

Brekhman II, Dardymov, IV. New Substances of Plant Origin which Increase Nonspecific Resist- ance. *Annual Review of Pharmacology,* 1969; 9.

Brown R, Gerberg P, Ramazanov Z. *Rhodiola Rosea;* A Phytomedicinal Overview. *Herbalgram,* 2002; 56:40–52.

Davidson JRT, et al. Effect of Hypericum Perforatum (St John's Wort) in Major Depressive Disorder: A Randomized Controlled Trial. *Journal of the American Medical Association*, 2002; 287: 1807–1814.

Dikasso D, Lemma H, Urga K, et al. Investigation on the Antibacterial Properties of Garlic (*Allium sativum*) on Pneumonia Causing Bacteria. *Ethiopian Med Journal*, 2002;40(3):241–249.

Giles J, Palat C, Chien S, et al. Evaluation of Echinacea for Treatment of the Common Cold. *Pharmacotherapy*, 2000; 20(6): 690–697.

Gubchenko PP, and Fruentov NK. Comparative Study of the Effectiveness of Eleutherococcus and Other Plant Adaptogens as Remedies for Increasing the Work Capacity of Flight Personnel. New Data on Eleutherococcus: Proceedings of the 2nd International Symposium on Eleutherococcus (Moscow, 1984). Vladivostok. Far East Academy of Sciences of the USSR, 1986, 240.

Hsing AW, Chokkalingam AP, Gao YT, et al. Allium Vegetables and Risk of Prostate Cancer: A Population-Based study. *Journal of the National Cancer Institute*, 2002; 94(21):1648–1651.

Kiso Y, Suzuki Y, Watanbe N, et al. Antihepatotoxic Principles of Curcuma Longa Rhizomes. *Planta Medical*, 1983; 49:185–187.

Le Bars P, Katz M, Berman N, et al. A Placebo-Controlled, Double-Blind, Randomized Trial of an Extract of Ginkgo Biloba for Dementia. *Journal of the American Medical Association*, 1997; 278: 16, 1327–1332.

Linde K, Ramirez G, Mulrow CD, et al. St John's Wort for Depression: An Overview and Meta-Analysis of Randomized Clinical Trials. *British Medical Journal*, 313; 1996:253–258.

Liu J, Manheimer E, Tsutani K, Gluud C. Medicinal Herbs for Hepatitis C Virus Infection: A Cochrane Hepatobiliary Systematic Review of Randomized Trials. *American Journal of Gastroenterol,* 2003; 98(3): 538–544.

Marks LS, Partin AW, Epstein JI, et al. Effects of a Saw Palmetto Herbal Blend in Men with Symptomatic Benign Prostatic Hyperplasia. *The Journal of Urology,* 2000; 163(5): 1451–1456.

Mix JA, Crews WD. A Double-Blind, Placebo-Controlled, Randomized Trial of Ginkgo Biloba Extract EGb 761 in a Sample of Cognitively Intact Older Adults: Neuropsychological Findings. *Human Experimental and Clinical Psychopharmacology,* 2002; 17: 267–277.

Ramirez-Bosca A, Soler A, Carrion-Guiterrez MA, et al. An Hydroalcoholic Extract of Curcuma Longa Lowers the Abnormally High Values of Human-Plasma Fibrinogen. *Mechanisms of Aging and Development,* 2000; 114:207–220.

Schoneberger D. The Influence of Immune-Stimulating Effects of Pressed Juice from Echinacea Purpurea on the Course and Severity of Colds. Results of a Double-Blind Study. *Forum Immunologie,* 1992; 8:2–12.

Schuppan D, Krebs A, Bauer M, Hahn EG. Hepatitis C and liver fibrosis. *Cell Death and Differentiation,* 2003; 10 Suppl 1:S59–67.

Sharifi AM, Darabi R, Akbarloo N. Investigation of Antihypertensive Mechanism of Garlic in 2K1C Hypertensive Rat. *Journal of Ethnopharmacology,* 2003; 86(2-3):219–224.

Sorenson H. A Double-Masked Study of the Effects of Ginseng on Cognitive Functions. *Current Therapeutic Research, Clinical and Experimental,* 1996; 57(12): 959–968.

Sotaneimi EA. Ginseng Therapy in Non-Insulin-Dependent Diabetic Patients. *Diabetes Care,* 1995; 18(10): 1373–1375.

Zhang Z, et al. Effect of Rhodiola on Preventing High Altitude Reactions: A Comparison of Cardiopulmonary Function in Villagers at Different Altitude Areas. *Journal of Chinese Materia Medica,* 1989; 14:47–50.

OTHER BOOKS AND RESOURCES

Balch, James and Balch, Phyllis. *Prescription for Herbal Healing.* New York: Avery, Penguin Putnam, 2002.

Blumenthal, Mark, et al. The Complete German Commission E Monographs: Therapeutic Guide to Herbal Medicines. Atlanta: Integrative Medicine Communications, 1998.

Blumenthal, Mark. *The ABC Clinical Guide to Herbs.* New York: Thieme Medical Publishers, 2003.

Brinker, Francis and Stodart, Nancy. *Herb Contraindications and Drug Interactions.* Sandy, OR: Eclectic Medical Publications, 2001.

Brown, Donald J. *Herbal Prescriptions for Health and Healing.* Twin Lakes, WI: Lotus Press, 2003.

Cass, Hyla. *St. John's Wort: Nature's Blues Buster.* New York: Avery, Penguin Putnam, 1998.

Cass, Hyla and Holford, Patrick. *Natural Highs: Supplements, Nutrition and Mind-Body Techniques to Help You Feel Good All the Time.* New York: Avery, Penguin Putnam, 2002.

Murray, Michael and Pizzorno, Joseph. *Encyclopedia of Natural Medicine.* Rocklin, CA: Prima Publishing, 1998.

Zand, Janet, Walton, Rachel, and Bob Rountree. *Smart Medicine for a Healthier Child: A Practical A-to-Z Reference to Natural and Conventional Treatments for Infants & Children.* New York: Avery, Penguin Putnam, 2003.

www.supplementinfo.org
A non-commercial informational website on the clinical use of various supplements.

National Center for Complementary and Alternative Medicine, National Institutes of Health (NIH)
http://nccam.nih.gov/about/advisory/capcam/
Searchable database of 180,000 bibliographic citations on complementary and alternative therapies extracted from MEDLINE.

GreatLife Magazine
Consumer magazine with articles on vitamins, minerals, herbs, and foods.
Available for free at many health and natural food stores.

Let's Live Magazine
Consumer magazine with emphasis on the health benefits of vitamins, minerals, and herbs.
Customer service:
1-800-676-4333
P.O. Box 74908
Los Angeles, CA 90004
Subscriptions: 12 issues per year, $19.95 in the U.S.; $31.95 outside the U.S.

Physical Magazine
Magazine oriented to body builders and other serious athletes.
Customer service:
1-800-676-4333

P.O. Box 74908
Los Angeles, CA 90004
Subscriptions: 12 issues per year, $19.95 in the U.S.; $31.95 outside the U.S.

The Nutrition Reporter™ newsletter
Monthly newsletter that summarizes recent medical research on vitamins, minerals, and herbs.
Customer service:
P.O. Box 30246
Tucson, AZ 85751-0246
e-mail: jack@thenutritionreporter.com
www.nutritionreporter.com
Subscriptions: $26 per year (12 issues) in the U.S.; $32 U.S. or $48 CNC for Canada; $38 for other countries.

INDEX